Renal Diet Cookbook For Beginners

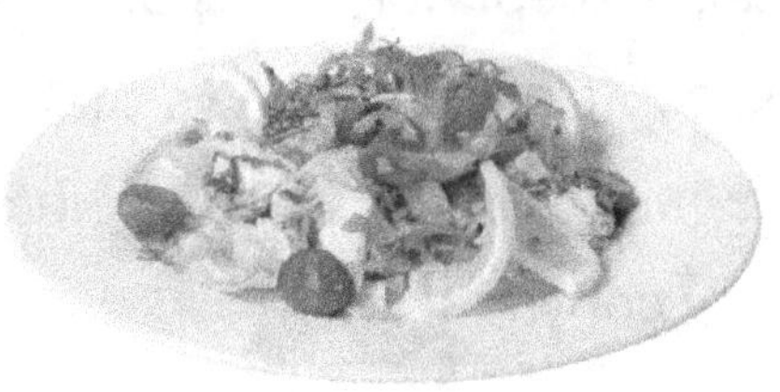

A Comprehensive Step By Step Guide To Managing Kidney Disease, Boosting Renal Health, And Preventing Dialysis through Healthy Diet

ALISON GUTIERREZ

Copyright © ALISON GUTIERREZ 2023

<u>Stress Management and Mental Well-being</u>
<u>CONCLUSION</u>

Introduction

Sarah, a middle-aged school teacher, faced a life-altering challenge. Diagnosed with chronic kidney disease, she was overwhelmed by fear and uncertainty. The prospect of dialysis loomed over her like a dark cloud, threatening to change her life forever. But amidst this storm, Sarah found a beacon of hope – a path to manage her condition and reclaim her health. It was through understanding her disease, adopting a renal-friendly diet, and the guidance of resources like this book that she turned her life around.

Kidney disease is often a silent invader, creeping up unnoticed until it reaches critical stages. It affects millions worldwide, altering the body's ability to filter waste and balance fluids. Sarah learned that understanding the nature of her disease was the first step towards empowerment. She discovered how her kidneys were struggling to perform their vital functions and why managing this condition was crucial for her overall health and well-being.

Diet, Sarah found, plays a pivotal role in managing kidney disease. She learned that certain foods could ease her kidney's workload, slowing the disease's progression and improving her quality of life. This book, much like the guide Sarah used, is filled with kidney-friendly recipes – each a blend of science, nutrition, and taste. It's not just about avoiding certain foods; it's about embracing a diet that nourishes and supports kidney health.

This comprehensive guide is more than just a cookbook. It's a companion for those walking the path Sarah did. It offers step-by-step guidance on how to manage kidney disease, boost renal health, and prevent the need for dialysis. Through delicious recipes and clear, compassionate advice, it provides the tools for readers to take control of their health, just as Sarah did.

Sarah's journey is a testament to the power of informed choices and dietary changes. From the despair of her diagnosis, she rose, empowered by knowledge and nourished by the right foods. Today, Sarah enjoys a life full of energy and hope, a life where kidney disease is a manageable part of her story, not the defining one. This book aims to offer the same hope and guidance to its readers, illuminating a path to better health and a brighter future.

Welcome to a journey of transformation and hope. If you're holding this book, you or a loved one might be facing the daunting world of kidney disease. It's a path filled with complexities and challenges, but also one where diet plays a pivotal role in managing and potentially transforming your health. This book is not just a collection of recipes; it's a beacon of hope and a guide to a healthier life.

Imagine a world where your diet becomes your ally in fighting against the progression of kidney disease. This is not a distant dream but a tangible reality that you can start working towards today. "Renal Cookbook for Beginners" is crafted with love and care, keeping in mind the unique needs of those newly diagnosed with kidney disease. It's more than just about what to eat and what to avoid; it's about understanding your body, the role of food, and how you can live a fulfilling life despite your diagnosis.

Kidney disease is often cloaked in mystery and fear. It's a condition that silently affects millions, gradually altering life in ways unimaginable. But within these pages lies the power to change that narrative. You'll find not just the science of renal diet but also stories of resilience and courage, of people just like you who have navigated these waters successfully.

Every chapter unfolds essential information in an easy-to-understand manner, removing the medical jargon that often clouds such discussions. From understanding your diagnosis to learning how different foods affect your kidneys, the book is a step-by-step guide designed to empower you. You'll learn how to prepare delicious meals that cater to your dietary needs, ensuring that every dish brings you closer to better kidney health.

This book isn't just about managing a condition; it's about redefining your life. It's a testament to the fact that a renal diet isn't a list of restrictions but a new canvas to paint your culinary skills on. It's a journey of discovery, of finding joy in the flavors that nourish you, and of celebrating the small victories along the way.

As you turn each page, remember that you're not alone in this journey. This book is a companion, a guide, and a friend that understands and supports you through every step of your renal health journey. Welcome to a new chapter in your life, one where you take control of your health, one delicious meal at a time.

Understanding Kidney Disease

Kidney disease, often a silent condition, can be a profound challenge to your health and lifestyle. It occurs when your kidneys can no longer effectively filter waste and excess fluids from your blood. This impairment can accumulate over time, due to factors like high blood pressure, diabetes, and genetic predispositions. Early stages often show no symptoms, making early detection difficult. Understanding this disease is crucial; it helps you recognize the signs and take proactive steps in managing your health. This knowledge empowers you to work closely with healthcare professionals to monitor and maintain your kidney function, potentially slowing the disease's progression.

The Importance of Diet in Managing Kidney Disease

Diet plays a critical role in managing kidney disease. As your kidneys' filtering ability diminishes, certain foods can exacerbate the condition, while others can help manage it. A diet tailored for kidney health focuses on reducing sodium, potassium, and phosphorus intake, which helps ease the kidneys' workload. It also involves controlling protein consumption to manage waste levels in the blood. Adhering to a renal-friendly diet can significantly slow the progression of kidney disease, alleviate symptoms, and improve your overall quality of life. It's about making informed choices that support your kidneys' health and well-being.

How This Book Can Help

This book is designed as a comprehensive guide to help you navigate the complexities of kidney disease and dietary management. It's structured to provide clear, actionable information and practical tips. You'll find detailed explanations of how different foods affect kidney health, along with a collection of kidney-friendly recipes. These recipes are not just healthy but also flavorful, ensuring that your diet remains a joy and not a chore. Additionally, the book offers guidance on lifestyle adjustments and coping strategies. It's a tool to educate, inspire, and support you in this journey towards better kidney health and improved quality of life.

Chapter 1: Basics of Renal Disease

Embarking on a journey towards understanding kidney disease is the first step in managing it effectively. This chapter aims to demystify the basics of renal disease, providing a solid foundation for anyone looking to deepen their understanding of this condition.

What is Kidney Disease?

Kidney disease, often referred to as renal disease, is a condition in which the kidneys are damaged and cannot filter blood as well as they should. This inefficiency can lead to a buildup of waste products in the body, which can have severe health implications. The kidneys are vital organs, performing crucial functions such as removing waste and excess fluid, maintaining the balance of electrolytes, and producing hormones that regulate blood pressure, red blood cell production, and bone health.

Stages of Kidney Disease

Kidney disease is typically categorized into five stages, based on the rate at which the kidneys filter blood (glomerular filtration rate, or GFR). These stages range from mild (stage 1) to complete kidney failure (stage 5). Early stages might have no symptoms, which makes the disease particularly insidious. As the disease progresses, symptoms such as fatigue, swollen limbs, difficulty concentrating, and poor appetite can develop. Understanding these stages is crucial for effective management and treatment.

Causes and Risk Factors

The causes of kidney disease are varied and include chronic conditions like diabetes and high blood pressure, which are among the most common causes. Other factors like heart disease, obesity, a family history of kidney failure, and age can increase the risk. Lifestyle factors, including smoking and excessive use of certain medications, can also contribute to the development of kidney disease.

Chapter 2: The Renal Diet Explained

In the quest to manage kidney disease effectively, understanding the renal diet is fundamental. This chapter delves into the principles of the renal diet, offering insight into the nutrients to monitor and providing guidance on foods to enjoy and avoid.

Principles of the Renal Diet

The renal diet is tailored to lessen the workload on the kidneys. This involves adjusting the intake of specific nutrients to prevent the accumulation of waste products in the blood. The key principles include controlling protein intake to reduce kidney strain, managing fluid intake to balance fluid levels in the body, and monitoring potassium, phosphorus, and sodium levels to maintain their delicate balance. Adhering to these principles helps in slowing the progression of kidney disease,

reducing the risk of complications, and enhancing overall well-being.

Nutrients to Monitor

1. Protein: Essential for tissue repair and immune function, but excessive intake can

burden the kidneys. The renal diet recommends moderate protein intake, focusing on high-quality sources.

2. Sodium: Excess sodium can lead to fluid retention and high blood pressure, worsening kidney damage. Limiting salt and avoiding high-sodium foods are crucial.

3. Potassium: While vital for muscle function and nerve health, impaired kidneys may not filter it properly, risking heart problems.

Monitoring and adjusting potassium intake is important.

4. Phosphorus: High levels can weaken bones in kidney disease patients. Limiting phosphorus-rich foods is essential to prevent bone complications.

Foods to Enjoy and Avoid

Enjoy: Fresh fruits and vegetables (mindful of potassium), lean meats, egg whites, garlic, herbs, and olive oil. Whole grains should be consumed in moderation.

Avoid: Processed foods high in sodium, dairy products rich in phosphorus, nuts, bananas, oranges, potatoes, and tomatoes due to high potassium. Red meat and other high-protein foods should be limited.

Chapter 3: Planning Your Renal Diet

Embarking on a renal diet requires careful planning and understanding. This chapter focuses on setting dietary goals, interpreting food labels accurately, and mastering portion control and meal planning. These skills are essential for anyone managing kidney disease through diet.

Setting Dietary Goals

The first step in adopting a renal diet is to set clear, achievable dietary goals. This involves understanding your specific nutritional needs based on the stage of your kidney disease, any other health conditions, and your overall health goals. Consultation with a healthcare provider or a dietitian can provide personalized guidance. Goals may include limiting certain nutrients like sodium, potassium, and phosphorus, ensuring adequate caloric intake, and maintaining a healthy weight. Setting these goals helps in creating a focused dietary plan that supports kidney health and overall well-being.

Reading Food Labels

Understanding food labels is crucial in adhering to a renal diet. Labels provide vital information about the nutritional content of foods, including their sodium, potassium, phosphorus, and protein levels. Learning to read and interpret these labels can empower you to make informed choices about what to include in your diet. Pay special attention to serving sizes, as they are key in managing nutrient intake.

Portion Control and Meal Planning

Effective portion control is vital in managing a renal diet. It helps in regulating the intake of nutrients that need to be monitored. Use measuring tools and visual cues to ensure accurate portion sizes.

Meal planning is another essential component. Planning meals in advance ensures that you have the right ingredients on hand to prepare kidney-friendly meals.

Chapter 4: Adapting Your Lifestyle

Successfully managing kidney disease isn't just about diet; it's about adopting a lifestyle that supports kidney health. This chapter explores how daily routines, fluid management, and dining out can be adjusted to suit the requirements of a renal diet.

Daily Routines and Kidney Health

Daily routines have a significant impact on kidney health. Regular physical activity, even moderate, can help manage blood pressure and sugar levels, critical factors in kidney disease. It's essential to integrate exercise into your daily routine, tailored to your individual capabilities and restrictions. Sleep is another crucial factor; adequate rest helps regulate kidney function and manage stress levels. Stress management techniques such as meditation, yoga, or simple breathing exercises can also be beneficial.

Managing Fluid Intake

Fluid balance is a key aspect of managing kidney disease. Depending on the stage of kidney disease and the individual's needs, fluid intake may need to be monitored closely. Excess fluid can strain the kidneys and lead to complications like hypertension and edema. It's important to understand your specific fluid requirements and develop strategies to manage intake, such as spacing out fluids throughout the day, avoiding foods with high water content, and recognizing signs of fluid overload.

Dining Out on a Renal Diet

Dining out while adhering to a renal diet can be challenging, but it's not impossible. It requires a bit of planning and assertiveness. Researching restaurants in advance, understanding menu items, and not hesitating to ask for modifications can make dining out a more enjoyable experience. Opt for dishes that are low in sodium, potassium, and phosphorus, and ask for sauces and dressings to be served on the side to control your intake.

Chapter 5: Renal Diet Recipes – Breakfast

Breakfast is the cornerstone of a daily diet, and when it comes to a renal diet, it's no different. This chapter focuses on easy and nutritious breakfast ideas, complete with ingredients, preparation methods, and cooking times, tailored for those on a renal diet.

Easy and Nutritious Breakfast Ideas

A renal diet breakfast balances the need for low sodium, potassium, and phosphorus while providing adequate energy and nutrition to start the day. Here are some ideas:

Savory Breakfast Options

1. Tofu Scramble: This plant-based alternative to traditional scrambled eggs uses tofu as the main ingredient. It's a lower-protein option that's kidney-friendly.

Ingredients: Firm tofu, turmeric, black pepper, and your choice of renal-friendly vegetables like bell peppers and zucchini.

Preparation: Crumble the tofu and sauté with spices and vegetables.

Cooking Time: Approximately 10-15 minutes.

2. **Avocado Toast with Kidney-Friendly Toppings:** A simple yet nutritious option that combines the healthy fats of avocado with whole grain bread.

Ingredients: Whole grain bread, ripe avocado, and toppings like cucumber or tomato slices.

Preparation: Mash the avocado and spread it on toasted bread, add toppings.

Cooking Time: About 5 minutes.

Sweet Breakfast Options

1. Berry and Chia Pudding: A delicious and nutritious start that's easy to prepare.

Ingredients: Chia seeds, almond milk, and fresh berries.

Preparation: Mix chia seeds with almond milk, let it sit overnight, then top with berries.

Cooking Time: Overnight soaking; minimal preparation in the morning.

2. **Renal-Friendly Oatmeal**: Oatmeal is versatile and can be dressed up with various toppings.

Ingredients: Rolled oats, water or almond milk, and toppings like apple slices or a sprinkle of cinnamon.

Preparation: Cook oats with liquid, add toppings.

Cooking Time: Approximately 10 minutes.

These breakfast ideas are not only renal-friendly but also satisfying and flavorful. They cater to different tastes and can be easily adapted to suit individual dietary needs. Remember, the key to a successful renal diet is not only in what you eat but also in how much and how often. Portion control and balancing nutrients are crucial for maintaining kidney health and overall well-being.

Chapter 6: Renal Diet Recipes - Lunch

Lunch on a renal diet doesn't have to be a challenge. This chapter focuses on healthy lunch options that cater to the specific nutritional needs of those with kidney disease. The recipes provided are low in sodium, potassium, and phosphorus, but still rich in flavor and nutrition.

Healthy Lunch Options

A renal-friendly lunch should be balanced, nutritious, and satisfying. Focus on incorporating a variety of vegetables, lean proteins, and whole grains that are lower in the nutrients you need to monitor.

Recipe 1: Grilled Chicken and Quinoa Salad
Ingredients: Skinless chicken breast, cooked quinoa, mixed greens (like lettuce and spinach), cherry tomatoes, cucumbers, and a dressing made with olive oil, lemon juice, and herbs.

Preparation: Grill the chicken breast and slice it. Toss the cooked quinoa and vegetables together, top with chicken and drizzle with dressing.

Cooking Time: Approximately 20-30 minutes. Instructions: Season the chicken lightly with herbs and grill until cooked. Combine the salad ingredients and top with grilled chicken. Mix the dressing ingredients and drizzle over the salad.

Recipe 2: Kidney-Friendly Tuna Salad Sandwich

Ingredients: Low-sodium canned tuna, light mayonnaise, diced celery, lettuce leaves, and whole wheat bread.

Preparation: Mix tuna with mayonnaise and celery. Assemble the sandwich with tuna mixture and lettuce.

Cooking Time: About 10 minutes.
Instructions: Drain the tuna and mix with a small amount of mayonnaise and diced celery. Spread on whole wheat bread and add lettuce leaves.

Recipe 3: Vegetable Stir-Fry with Brown Rice

Ingredients: A variety of kidney-friendly vegetables like bell peppers, carrots, and zucchini, brown rice, low-sodium soy sauce, garlic, and ginger.

Preparation: Cook the brown rice as directed. Stir-fry the vegetables in a pan with a bit of oil, garlic, and ginger.

Cooking Time: Rice (according to package instructions), vegetables (10-15 minutes).

Instructions: Start by cooking the brown rice. In a separate pan, sauté the vegetables with garlic and ginger until they are tender-crisp. Add a splash of low-sodium soy sauce for flavor. Serve the stir-fry over the cooked rice.

These lunch recipes are designed to be kidney-friendly, focusing on limiting certain nutrients while still providing a balanced and flavorful meal. Remember, portion control is key in managing a renal diet.

Chapter 7: Dinner Recipes: Ingredients, Preparation, Cooking Time, and Instructions

1. Creamy Butternut Squash Soup

Ingredients:
1 butternut squash
1 onion
Low-sodium vegetable broth
A touch of nutmeg
Fresh parsley (for garnish)

Preparation & Cooking Time:
- Roast squash and onion, then blend with vegetable broth.
- Simmer for 15 minutes.
- Season with a pinch of nutmeg.
- Garnish with fresh parsley.

2. Balsamic Glazed Chicken Breast

Ingredients:
- Skinless, boneless chicken breasts
- Low-sodium balsamic vinegar
- Garlic cloves
- Fresh rosemary
- Olive oil

Preparation & Cooking Time:
- Marinate chicken in balsamic vinegar, garlic, and rosemary.
- Sear chicken in olive oil.
- Glaze with balsamic reduction.
- Bake until tender and juicy.

3. Quinoa and Vegetable Stir-Fry

Ingredients:
- Quinoa
- Mixed stir-fry vegetables (broccoli, bell peppers, snap peas)
- Low-sodium soy sauce
- Garlic and ginger
- Sesame oil

Preparation & Cooking Time:
- Cook quinoa according to package instructions.
- Sauté garlic and ginger.
- Stir-fry vegetables.
- Toss with quinoa, soy sauce, and a drizzle of sesame oil.

These recipes represent just a taste of the culinary delights awaiting you. Each dish is crafted with your kidney health in mind, providing a harmony of flavors while managing the critical aspects of a renal diet. We'll guide you through the step-by-step process, ensuring that you not only prepare nourishing meals but also develop confidence in your culinary skills.

As you explore these recipes, you'll find that mastering the renal diet isn't just about managing kidney disease; it's about savoring a world of flavors, nourishing your body, and gaining control of your health.

Chapter 8: Snacks and Beverages

In Chapter 8, we explore the delightful world of snacks and beverages, a realm where kidney-conscious choices play a pivotal role in maintaining and improving kidney health. This chapter is your gateway to mastering these essential components of the renal diet, and it's divided into three sections:

Kidney-Friendly Snacks

Snacking can be a joyous part of life, even on a renal diet. Here, we'll embark on a journey to discover snacks that are not only delicious but also tailored to support your kidney health. These snacks are thoughtfully chosen to be low in phosphorus, potassium, and sodium, making them perfect for those with kidney disease. From satisfying homemade trail mix to crunchy cucumber and carrot sticks with a yogurt dip, you'll find options that tantalize your taste buds while respecting your dietary restrictions.

Safe Beverages and Drinks

Proper hydration is a cornerstone of kidney health, and your beverage choices matter. This section guides you through selecting beverages that keep you well-hydrated while aligning with your renal diet goals. We'll explore the best choices to manage phosphorus and potassium levels, ensuring your drinks contribute positively to your overall well-being.

Snack and Beverage Recipes: Ingredients, Preparation, Cooking Time, and Instructions

To empower you with practical guidance, we've curated a collection of snack and beverage recipes. Each recipe comes complete with a detailed list of ingredients, step-by-step preparation instructions, estimated cooking times, and practical tips to make the process effortless.

1. **Nutty Banana Smoothie**

Ingredients:
- Ripe bananas

- Almond milk
- Natural almond butter
- A sprinkle of cinnamon

Preparation:
- Blend bananas, almond milk, and almond butter until smooth.
- Sprinkle with a dash of cinnamon.

Cooking Time:
- 5 minutes

2. **Mediterranean Chickpea Salad**

Ingredients:
- Chickpeas
- Cherry tomatoes
- Cucumber
- Red onion
- Feta cheese (optional)
- Olive oil and lemon juice dressing

Preparation:
- Combine chickpeas, cherry tomatoes, cucumber, and red onion.
- Add optional feta cheese if desired.
- Drizzle with olive oil and lemon juice dressing.

Kidney-Friendly Snacks

Snacks play an important role in the renal diet by providing nutrients between meals. Some healthy, kidney-friendly snacks include:

- Fresh fruits like apples, blueberries, grapes, and strawberries
- Vegetables sticks with hummus or guacamole
- A small handful of unsalted nuts or seeds
- Rice cakes or crackers with peanut butter or cheese
- Plain yogurt mixed with fruit
- Hard-boiled eggs
- Air-popped popcorn

Focus on snacks that provide fiber, vitamins, and minerals while being low in sodium, potassium, and phosphorus. Check food labels and choose options with less than 200mg sodium per serving.

Safe Beverages and Drinks

Staying hydrated is important when following a renal diet. Some kidney-friendly beverage options include:

- Water - the best option, add lemon or lime for flavor
- Unsweetened cranberry juice
- Black coffee
- Unsweetened tea
- Low-potassium vegetable juices like carrot juice

Avoid sweetened beverages, sports drinks, soda, coconut water, and alcohol as these can further strain the kidneys.

Snack and Beverage Recipes

Try these simple yet delicious recipes:

Strawberry Infused Water
Ingredients: 2 cups water, 1 cup strawberries
Instructions: Add water and strawberries to a pitcher. Refrigerate for at least 2 hours before serving.

Roasted Chickpeas
Ingredients: 1 15oz can chickpeas, drained and rinsed; 1 tsp olive oil; 1 tsp chili powder; 1/2 tsp garlic powder; 1/2 tsp paprika

Instructions: Toss chickpeas with oil and spices. Roast at 400°F for 30 minutes, shaking halfway.

Iced Coffee

Ingredients: 1 cup cold brewed coffee, 1/4 cup low-fat milk
Instructions: Stir milk into coffee and serve over ice.

These recipes are your companions on the journey to savoring snacks and beverages that not only gratify your palate but also uphold your kidney health. The instructions provided ensure that your culinary endeavors are as smooth and enjoyable as possible. Enjoy this flavorful exploration of managing kidney disease through diet, one snack and sip at a time.

Chapter 12: Beyond Diet – Holistic Kidney Care

In our journey towards holistic kidney care, we've explored the significance of a well-balanced diet in maintaining kidney health. But, to truly achieve a holistic approach, we need to look beyond diet and consider other vital aspects of our lifestyle that impact our kidneys. In this chapter, we delve into two crucial elements: Exercise and Kidney Health, and Stress Management and Mental Well-being.

Exercise and Kidney Health

Physical activity is a cornerstone of a healthy lifestyle, and its benefits extend to kidney health. Regular exercise can contribute significantly to the prevention of kidney problems and the management of existing kidney conditions. Here's how:

1. **Improved Blood Pressure Control**: High blood pressure is a leading cause of kidney disease. Engaging in regular physical activity

helps lower blood pressure, reducing the strain on the kidneys and the risk of kidney damage.

2. **Enhanced Cardiovascular Health:** A strong heart and healthy blood vessels are essential for optimal kidney function. Exercise promotes cardiovascular health, ensuring that your kidneys receive an adequate blood supply.

3. **Weight Management:** Obesity is a risk factor for kidney disease. Exercise plays a pivotal role in weight management, helping to maintain a healthy body weight and reduce the risk of kidney problems.

4. **Blood Sugar Regulation:** Regular physical activity can improve insulin sensitivity and help regulate blood sugar levels. This is particularly important for individuals with diabetes, as uncontrolled diabetes can lead to kidney complications.

5. **Strengthening Immune Function:** Exercise boosts the immune system, which is crucial for preventing kidney infections and maintaining overall kidney health.

However, it's essential to strike a balance. Intense or excessive exercise can sometimes lead to muscle breakdown, releasing waste products that the kidneys must filter. Therefore, consult with a healthcare provider to develop an exercise plan tailored to your specific needs and limitations.

Stress Management and Mental Well-being

The connection between stress and kidney health is not widely known, but it's significant. Chronic stress can take a toll on the body, including the kidneys. Here's why addressing stress and nurturing mental well-being is integral to holistic kidney care:

1. **Blood Pressure:** Stress triggers the release of stress hormones, which can elevate blood pressure. Prolonged high blood pressure can damage the kidneys over time.

2. **Inflammation**: Chronic stress is linked to increased inflammation in the body, which can negatively impact kidney function and contribute to kidney disease.

3. **Adherence to Treatment:** Managing a kidney condition often involves strict dietary restrictions and medication. Stress can make it more challenging to adhere to these treatment plans, potentially worsening kidney health.

4. **Quality of Life:** Kidney disease can be physically and emotionally taxing. Stress management techniques, such as mindfulness, meditation, and therapy, can improve the overall quality of life for individuals with kidney conditions.

5. **Preventive Measures:** Reducing stress and promoting mental well-being can help prevent the development of kidney problems in the first place, as stress is a known risk factor.

CONCLUSION

Incorporating stress-reduction strategies and seeking professional help when needed can be as crucial to kidney health as dietary choices. Remember that taking care of your mental well-being is not a luxury but an essential part of a holistic approach to kidney care.

In the pages of "Renal Diet Cookbook for Beginners," we've embarked on a transformative journey towards managing kidney disease, nurturing renal health, and safeguarding against the need for dialysis through the power of a wholesome diet. With each chapter, we've uncovered the intricate interplay between nutrition, kidney function, and overall well-being. It's a journey that has taken us from understanding the fundamentals of renal disease to crafting delicious and kidney-friendly meals, and finally, to embracing a holistic approach to kidney care.

Our exploration began by demystifying the complexities of kidney disease, shedding light on its stages, causes, and risk factors. Armed with this knowledge, we ventured into the heart of the renal diet, unraveling its principles and the nutrients that require careful monitoring. We learned how to set dietary goals, decipher food labels, and master portion control and meal planning.

Through every chapter, we navigated the intricacies of daily routines, fluid management, and the art of dining out while adhering to our dietary restrictions. Our culinary journey continued as we explored breakfast, lunch, and dinner recipes that not only tantalize the taste buds but also prioritize kidney health.

We are introduced to the world of kidney-friendly snacks and beverages, ensuring that our choices between meals align with our renal diet goals. We discovered that snacks need not be bland, and beverages can be both refreshing and kidney-conscious.

As we reached the final chapters, we delved into holistic kidney care, acknowledging the significance of exercise, stress management, and mental well-being in our quest for optimal health. We realized that a well-rounded approach to kidney care extends beyond diet alone.

In conclusion, "Renal Diet Cookbook for Beginners" is more than just a cookbook; it's a comprehensive guide to transforming lives. It empowers us to take control of our health, one delicious meal at a time, and equips us with the knowledge and tools needed to navigate the challenges of kidney disease with confidence.

As we embrace a new way of eating and living, let this book be our constant companion, offering guidance, inspiration, and hope. Together, we can nurture our kidneys, safeguard our health, and embark on a brighter, healthier future. This journey is a testament to the power of informed choices, nourishing foods, and the unwavering spirit of those committed to their kidney health. Welcome to a life where kidney disease is a manageable part of our story, not the defining one.